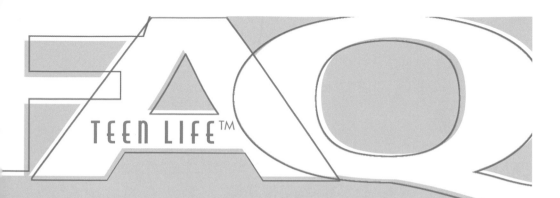

TEEN LIFE™

FREQUENTLY ASKED QUESTIONS ABOUT

Diabetes

Judith Levin

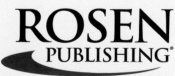

ROSEN
PUBLISHING®
New York

To all teens who live with the challenge of diabetes

Published in 2007 by The Rosen Publishing Group, Inc.
29 East 21st Street, New York, NY 10010

Library of Congress Cataloging-in-Publication Data

Levin, Judith, 1956–
Frequently asked questions about diabetes / by Judith Levin.—1st ed.
p. cm.—(FAQ: teen life)
Includes bibliographical references.
ISBN-13: 978-1-4042-0961-9
ISBN-10: 1-4042-0961-1 (library binding)
1. Diabetes—Popular works. I. Title.
RC660.4.L48 2007
616.4'62—dc22

2006021519

Manufactured in the United States of America

Contents

Introduction

More and more, people with diabetes are doing things that doctors used to say were impossible. "Your career is over," a doctor told cross-country skier Kris Freeman when he was diagnosed with diabetes at age nineteen. Freeman went on to compete in the 2006 Olympics.

A diagnosis of diabetes wouldn't be anyone's first choice of news from his or her doctor. Yet, by understanding what diabetes is and how to live with it, people with the disease are discovering they can do pretty much whatever they want with their lives.

If you've just been told that you have diabetes, you may feel a little like Mario, who was diagnosed with it when he was ten. His uncle, meaning to encourage him, told him the inspiring story of someone with diabetes who had climbed Mount Everest. Already overwhelmed, Mario yelled, "You mean I have to climb Mount Everest, too?!" OK, so you may not feel like climbing Mount Everest right now, but you do need to believe that your life is not over. If you've had diabetes since you were a kid, then you need to know that puberty may make it harder to control. If you're reading this because a friend or family member has diabetes, then you can find out what this disease is all about and how to help in an emergency.

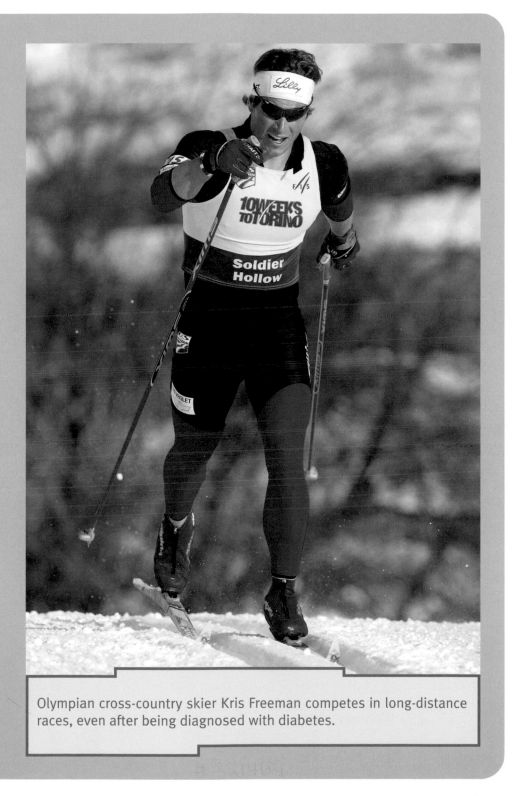

Olympian cross-country skier Kris Freeman competes in long-distance races, even after being diagnosed with diabetes.

KELLY'S STORY

When Kelly goes skydiving, she tucks jelly beans under her jumpsuit. On white-water rafting trips, she zips mints in waterproof pouches under her flotation vest. For underground cave explorations, she gives the group leader her emergency kit.

After Kelly was diagnosed with diabetes at age fourteen, she cried and yelled and kicked a hole in her bedroom wall. This can't be happening to me, she thought.

Her doctor told her, "We'll get this under control. I know you're overwhelmed, but you're going to be able to handle it."

Yeah, right. How did he know? she thought.

For months, Kelly refused to tell anyone but her best friend what she was going through. She didn't want pity, and she didn't want people treating her differently. Even after Kelly had gotten — sort of — used to having diabetes in her life, she still felt "different" and very alone.

Her mom made her talk to somebody on her support team about her frustrations. Her diabetes educator then put her in touch with a group of other teens with diabetes. Some of them had just been diagnosed; some had been living with diabetes since they were little. "It doesn't have to define me," one guy told her. "It's only one part of my life — an annoying part — but it isn't the most important thing about me."

Kelly decided that she wasn't going to let some stupid disease ruin her life. "I don't know if I ever would have discovered adventure sports if I hadn't been diagnosed," she says now, ten years later.

"Having the diagnosis made me want to push myself harder and see what I could do."

Of course, Kelly, like everyone else who has diabetes, longs for a cure or even a week off from her careful monitoring of her food intake, blood sugar levels, and ketones. But all that attention is what keeps her healthy and strong enough to try a new sport when she wants to—and it makes it very likely that she will be able to keep doing the things she loves for many more years.

Modern technology helps Kelly keep her diabetes under control, but so does her take-charge attitude. "It takes planning everything," she says, "and I get sick of it. I hated losing the spontaneity to be able to do whatever I want and leave the house without checking that I had all my supplies. My friends don't have to do that and I wish I didn't, but getting careless isn't worth it. I wind up feeling crummy, and I know I could wind up paying for it later."

WHAT IS DIABETES?

Diabetes is a disease in which the body either does not produce, or does not properly use, insulin. Insulin is a hormone that helps the body change food into energy. The stomach and small intestine convert the carbohydrates we eat into the body's main fuel, glucose, a kind of sugar. When released into the bloodstream as blood sugar, glucose circulates through the body and feeds the cells.

The two most common forms of diabetes are type I and type II. In type I diabetes, the body can't produce any insulin. When a person has type II diabetes, he or she can't produce enough insulin, can't use it efficiently, or both.

Type I Diabetes

Type I diabetes accounts for about 5 to 10 percent of diabetes cases in the United States.

Pancreas Anatomy

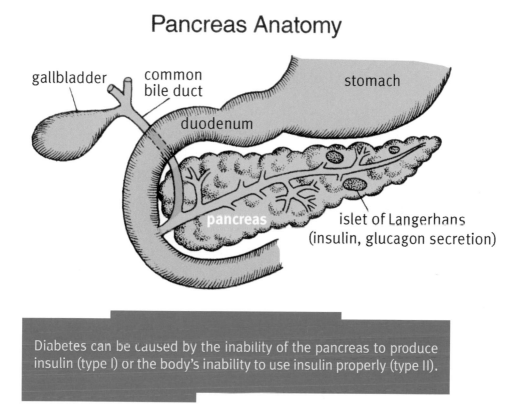

gallbladder

common
bile duct

stomach

duodenum

pancreas

islet of Langerhans
(insulin, glucagon secretion)

Diabetes can be caused by the inability of the pancreas to produce insulin (type I) or the body's inability to use insulin properly (type II).

Type I was once called juvenile diabetes, but because adults develop it, too, this term is no longer used. In type I diabetes, the beta cells in the pancreas (a small organ behind the stomach) don't produce insulin, even though they should. In the body of someone with type I diabetes, there is no insulin, and as a result, sugar builds up in the bloodstream. The starving cells cause the body to burn fat for energy, releasing toxic ketone bodies into the blood. Because people with type I diabetes must always take insulin, it also used to be called insulin-dependent diabetes.

Type I diabetes is an autoimmune disease. In autoimmune diseases, the body's defense systems go on a seek-and-destroy mission of something that is part of the body, rather than confining their attentions to intruding infections, which is what they are supposed to be doing. Researchers believe that some kind of trigger—probably a virus—has caused the white blood cells to attack the beta cells in the pancreas in a person with type I diabetes. Type I diabetes is caused by an inherited vulnerability to it—it's in a person's genes. However, the chance of a person with type I diabetes passing the disease on to his or her children is relatively small.

Type II Diabetes

In type II diabetes, once known as noninsulin-dependent diabetes, the body either cannot use its insulin properly or it can't produce enough of it. About 90 percent of the people with diabetes have type II, but until recently nearly all those people were older adults. Ten years ago, it wouldn't even be discussed as a possibility for teens. But type II is dramatically on the rise among people of all ages, including teens and even young children.

The Causes

Researchers believe people are developing type II diabetes because of poor eating habits and because they prefer sitting on the couch watching TV or hunching over a keyboard or Gameboy to exercising. Fast food is engineered to be tasty, but it is, of course, high in fats and carbohydrates. Our bodies need

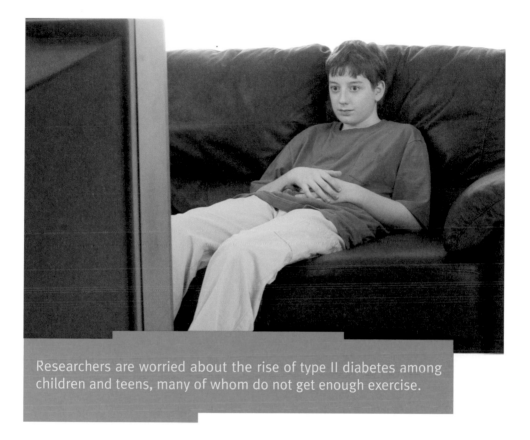

Researchers are worried about the rise of type II diabetes among children and teens, many of whom do not get enough exercise.

more insulin to convert the carbs into glucose. The bigger we are, the more insulin we need. Being overweight causes insulin resistance. Exercise lowers blood sugar and burns calories. It also increases muscle, which should be absorbing 70 to 90 percent of our blood sugar. Schools with tight budgets are often cutting gym class. Some city schools don't even have playgrounds.

Type II diabetes is caused in part by an inherited vulnerability, but also by too little exercise and too many calories: it's in your genes, but also in your jeans. The upside is that type II diabetes can often be avoided or controlled through lifestyle changes.

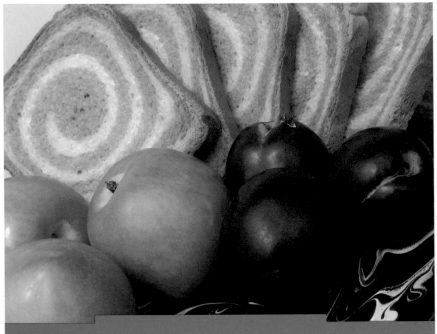

A healthful diet—one including foods from all the major food groups—will help prevent some teens and adults from developing type II diabetes.

Who Gets Type II Diabetes?

Some racial and ethnic groups are particularly vulnerable to type II diabetes. Twice as many African Americans and Latinos get type II than Caucasians. (More Caucasians than African Americans get type I.) Asian Americans and people from the Pacific Islands can get type II without putting on much extra weight. Researchers believe that more people in these groups have a "thrifty gene": ancestors who hunted and farmed had a gene that allowed them to put weight on more easily. Getting fatter was seen as a good thing. It meant that they were less likely to starve during a time of illness or food shortages.

The modern diet makes it too easy to gain weight. Kids and teens in poor families are particularly at risk because they are less likely to see a doctor regularly, especially when they don't seem to be sick. Also, type II diabetes can be easier to ignore— for a while anyway—than type I. There may not be symptoms, but in reality, the body is being damaged.

Rare Types of Diabetes

Other types of diabetes include gestational diabetes, which is experienced temporarily by about 1 to 4 percent of pregnant women. Diabetes caused by damage to the pancreas, infections, or as a side effect of some medicines are other forms.

WHAT ARE THE SYMPTOMS OF DIABETES?

High blood sugar can happen as a result of diabetes but it is not the cause. People with diabetes can have a lot of or no symptoms, and their symptoms can be very severe or relatively mild. Type II diabetes in particular can be nearly symptom-free for a long time. Researchers estimate that about a third of people who have type II diabetes don't know it and may go seven to ten years without a diagnosis. Yet, in this time, they may have already developed dangerous and irreversible complications. If you have symptoms of diabetes, or are at high risk of getting it, you should be tested for it. People who are at high risk for developing type II diabetes typically have close family members with the disease, are in a racial or ethnic group in which diabetes cases are high, or have high blood pressure or high blood cholesterol. Warning signs of both types include:

- Having to urinate often
- Having a dry mouth and being really thirsty all of the time
- Losing weight, even though you're eating normally or even eating a lot
- Extreme hunger
- Blurry vision
- Numbness or tingling in the hands or feet
- Feeling tired or weak
- Very dry skin or skin infections
- Cuts and scratches healing slowly

These symptoms may be less pronounced in someone with type II diabetes, and the sufferer won't lose weight without effort. In fact, he or she may even gain weight. The skin of somebody with type II diabetes may be dry and itchy, and there is sometimes a darkening of the skin around the neck, armpits, and groin, which can be a sign of insulin resistance.

A Biological Look at the Symptoms

The symptoms of diabetes make sense if you understand what the body is trying to cope with. Since cells can't use the carbs that a person with diabetes is eating, sugar builds up in the blood. The kidneys try to get rid of it by producing more urine to flush the sugar out of the body. They even suck water out of the body's tissues, dehydrating them—causing dry skin and a dry mouth and an incredible thirst. (A small child is sometimes diagnosed after parents tell the doctor that their kid has been

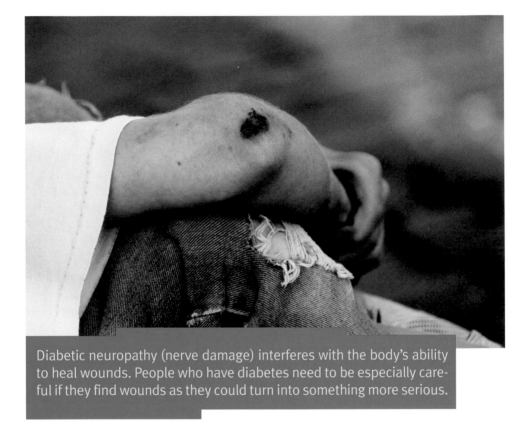

Diabetic neuropathy (nerve damage) interferes with the body's ability to heal wounds. People who have diabetes need to be especially careful if they find wounds as they could turn into something more serious.

drinking his or her bathwater.) Dehydration can also lead to blurry vision.

Type I

If the body's cells are starving because they're not getting the glucose they need, the body is going to try to feed them another way: it's going to burn protein and body fat. As fat breaks down, it releases acids called ketones. Some of these are cleared out of your system by the frequent urination, but the ketones can start to build up and poison you. (It's called ketoacidosis.) Even with

People with diabetes can suffer from infections of wounds on their feet. Without proper care, infections can become dangerous and might require amputations.

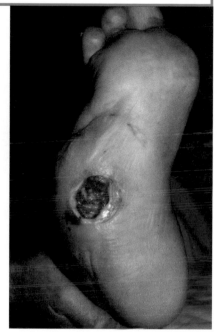

your body burning fat, your cells are starving. They're sending "feed me" signals that you experience as hunger. Even with the extra food, your cells still aren't getting the energy they need, so you may feel weak.

High blood sugar levels can also damage nerves. Your hands and feet may tingle, or you might get leg cramps. Finally, the high sugar levels feed bacteria and interfere with your white blood cells, so cuts may be slower to heal and skin infections may develop easily. Your body is doing the best it can, but it needs help!

Complications

Complications from improperly cared-for type I and II diabetes are real and scary. People with type I can have reactions if they let their blood sugar go too low or too high. However, these complications can take a few years or decades to develop due to blood sugar levels that aren't immediately dangerous. That's the

Blood vessel damage to the retina of the eye (retinopathy) can cause vision problems or even blindness in people with diabetes.

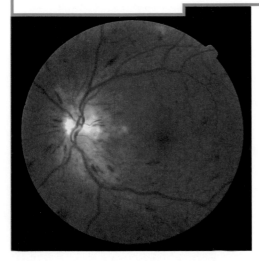

problem: they won't make you unconscious, but they damage your body and your internal organs in a major way. Years of high blood sugar can result in long-term complications.

Nerve and Blood Vessel Damage

High levels of blood sugar damage the nerves, probably by weakening the capillaries (tiny blood vessels) that bring blood to the nerves to nourish them. This damage, called diabetic neuropathy, can be mild or it can be severe and disabling.

Neuropathy can affect the muscles, causing weakness. It can interfere with a man's ability to have an erection. Often, the damage takes the form of tingling, pain, or numbness in the feet. Someone with nerve damage to the feet may not realize he or she has a cut or scratch until it becomes infected. Because diabetes also interferes with the body's ability to heal wounds, dangerous foot infections can happen in people with the condition. Amputations are not unusual.

The good news is that most of this can be prevented. You're going to want to keep that blood sugar in range and take good care of your feet, washing and drying them carefully and checking for cuts, even tiny ones, in good light.

The eyes are also vulnerable to blood vessel damage in the retina, located at the back of the eyes. Six out of ten people with type II develop vision problems, but this statistic is misleading because it is based on problems people experience after twenty years of living with the disease. As increasing numbers of young people are diagnosed with type II diabetes, more will be living with the disease for more than twenty years. Great strides have been made in the past two decades, and many diabetes-related eye problems can now be treated.

Kidney Damage

The kidneys remove waste from our blood. This waste is then flushed out of our bodies when we urinate. Dealing with too much glucose over a period of years can damage the kidneys. They work less, or stop working completely. People whose kidneys have stopped working need to go for dialysis several times a week. During dialysis, they are hooked up to a machine that filters the blood. Some people may even need a new kidney—a transplant. Again, prevention is the key, with daily blood sugar management and annual screenings for early detection and treatment.

Heart and Blood Vessel Disease

Teens don't have to worry about having heart attacks from their diabetes, but the disease does increase their chances of having problems later on by damaging their arteries. Damaged arteries can cause heart attacks, strokes, and high blood pressure.

three

HOW IS DIABETES DIAGNOSED?

Diabetes has been recognized since ancient times. The full name of the disease is diabetes mellitus. In Greek, *diabetes* means "to siphon" or "to suck out." It is believed to have been named around 230 BC by a Greek physician who hypothesized that the body of someone with diabetes was melting down and turning into urine. *Mellitus* is the Latin word for "honey" and refers to the sugar in the urine of someone who has diabetes. Until the twentieth century, doctors and healers routinely smelled and tasted a patient's urine as part of their diagnoses. They found that people with diabetes had sweet pee. (Gross, but they had to go by what they could observe. The ancient Chinese diagnosed diabetes by waiting to see if ants were attracted to a bowl of the patient's urine.) Doctors also observed that the breath of these patients smelled fruity. This was not a healthy

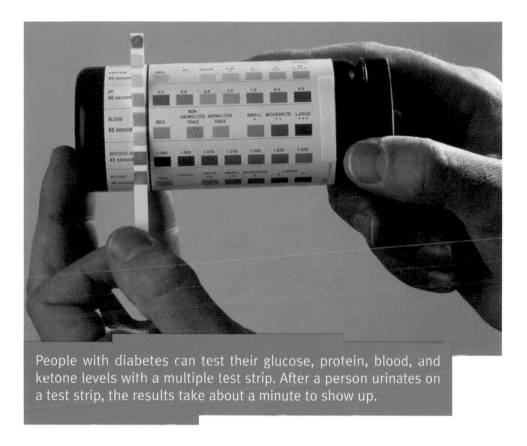

People with diabetes can test their glucose, protein, blood, and ketone levels with a multiple test strip. After a person urinates on a test strip, the results take about a minute to show up.

sign and it still isn't, as it indicates that ketones have built up in the blood. Modern science is more precise, but the general idea is the same: the doctor is looking for signs of too much sugar in the blood.

Modern Screening Tests

If one drop of your blood is tested and shows that your blood sugar is too high, your doctor will order a diagnostic test. There are various ways of testing for diabetes.

Ten Great Questions to Ask if You Have Diabetes

1 How do I know when I need to call my doctor or go to an emergency room?

2 Should I get a pump?

3 Whom can I talk to about my diabetes?

4 How do I know how different foods will affect my blood sugar level?

5 Whom do I need to tell that I have diabetes? What should I tell my friends?

6 Can I still play sports?

7 Will I be able to have children? Will they have diabetes, too?

8 Why are my blood sugar levels high some days, even though I'm being careful?

9 Can I drive? How do I know what activities I can do safely?

10 What should I carry with me for emergencies?

Fasting Plasma Glucose Test

"Fasting" means that the person doesn't eat or drink anything, except water, for at least eight hours before the test. Different foods and amounts of food affect blood sugar in different ways, so this test shows what the body is doing without the doctor having to consider those variables. The doctor takes a sample of blood for analysis and measures the amount of glucose in the plasma. Plasma is the clear yellowish part of the blood that carries red and white blood cells. It also carries glucose.

Someone without diabetes will have a fasting plasma glucose level that is between 70 and 99 milligrams per deciliter. A milligram is 1/1,000 of a gram (a small paper clip weighs about a gram). A deciliter is 1/10 of a liter. If a person's blood has more than 100 milligrams of glucose per deciliter of plasma, then that person is not using glucose well. If the fasting blood glucose level is above 126 mg/dL, and it remains that high when tested on another day, then the patient will be diagnosed with diabetes. A blood sugar level between 100 and 125 mg/dL is considered pre-diabetic, which means a person is at risk of developing the disease.

One drop of blood placed on a chemically coated strip inserted into a glucometer is enough to show whether a person's blood sugar level is "in range."

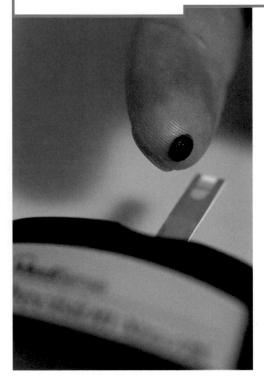

Research shows that paying attention to diet, activity, and weight can help to prevent or delay the onset of type II.

Oral Glucose Tolerance Test

American Diabetes Association guidelines say that the results of two fasting glucose tests are enough to diagnose diabetes. Some doctors will also use an oral glucose tolerance test, however.

This test is given after an eight-hour or overnight fast. The doctor takes a blood sample to get a fasting glucose level. Then the patient drinks a very sweet glucose liquid and gets his or her blood tested again at thirty-minute intervals for two hours.

If someone has a healthy amount of insulin, and he or she can use that insulin properly, then the blood sugar level rises soon after the glucose drink but returns to normal. That person's insulin has caused the cells to absorb the glucose. In the body of someone who has diabetes, the glucose level in the bloodstream

Gary Hall Jr., Olympic medalist in swimming, tests his blood ten to twelve times a day to be sure he is keeping his type I diabetes under control.

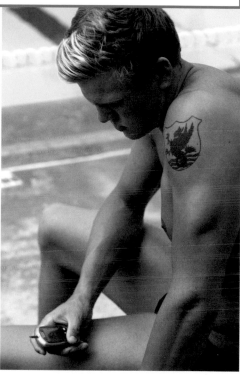

goes higher and stays high for much longer. A level above 200 mg/dL two hours after a drink containing 3 ounces (85 grams) of glucose indicates diabetes.

Glycosylated Hemoglobin Test

If a person has been diagnosed with diabetes, a doctor may order the glycosylated hemo- globin test, which is also known as the hemoglobin A1c. It is a measure of a person's average blood sugar level over the last two to three months, as indicated by the amount of sugar on the red blood cells. (A red blood cell lives about two to three months.)

For someone with diabetes, the test is given two to four times a year. It gives a rough average of what a person's blood sugar level has been over that time. Once somebody's diabetes is under control, the result will, ideally, be about the same as it would be for someone without the disease.

four

HOW IS DIABETES TREATED?

Unfortunately, there is still no cure for diabetes (except for a pancreas transplant for type I). Diabetes treatment is based on keeping blood sugar (glucose) in as normal a range as possible. For someone with type I diabetes, treatment includes the injection of insulin. For both types I and II, it may include changing what you eat and getting more exercise. Someone with type II may or may not need injected insulin but may be given pills that help the body use its own insulin better.

Blood Sugar Levels

For people with diabetes, controlling their blood sugar is the most important thing, so they have to be able to measure it. This is done by placing a test strip into a blood glucose meter and pricking the finger with a lancet and putting one drop of blood on the chemically treated test strip. The monitor gives a number that tells whether the blood sugar is high, low, or within range. Some monitors will record this information and allow a person to download it into a computer, and some will store it so that its user can later write it down. This information partly tells if a person is taking the right amount and kind of insulin, but over time it shows how daily life—popcorn overload, baseball practice, math homework, or a fight with a friend—affects the blood sugar level. That's why keeping a record of blood glucose readings is important. It helps people with diabetes to manage their diabetes and to detect patterns that will allow them to spend more time "in range." This might be between 70 and 100 mg/dL before meals and between 100 and 140 mg/dL at bedtime. Work with your diabetes support team to determine blood sugar goals that are best for you.

As blood sugar tests have become easier to do, blood sugar has become easier to control. Research shows that staying in range really cuts down on complications, and so people with diabetes are starting to test their blood more often. Generally, three or four times a day (in the morning and before meals) is a minimum for someone with type I, but testing more often allows for better control of blood sugar. A doctor, diabetes educator (someone trained in helping people manage day-to-day diabetes treatment and concerns), and the patient will work out how often and when tests are needed.

People will usually experience symptoms when their blood sugar is low (hypoglycemia) or high (hyperglycemia). Some people, however, do not get the early-warning symptoms of low blood sugar, which are:

- Sweating
- Shakiness
- Extreme hunger
- Dizziness
- Weakness
- Irritability/crankiness
- Cold, clammy skin
- Fast heartbeat
- Nausea
- Headache

If their blood sugar is allowed to continue to drop, those with diabetes will feel and appear confused and sleepy. They may seem drunk—uncoordinated and slurring their words. Beyond that point, they may have convulsions or become unconscious and die.

A quick tip for people with diabetes and their friends and family: if someone's blood sugar gets low, he or she needs fast-acting carbs immediately. Glucose tablets are sold in drugstores and some people with diabetes carry them, but half a cup of fruit juice, five pieces of hard candy, a cup of milk, or one-third of a can of (nondiet) soda will do. If someone you're with has very low blood sugar, he or she may be confused, panicky, or cranky. Getting those carbs into him or her could be literally a matter of life and death.

High Blood Sugar (Hyperglycemia)

Someone with high blood sugar may have symptoms similar to diabetes, since the symptoms of diabetes include high blood

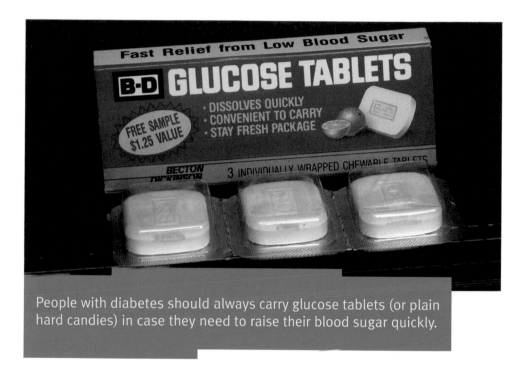

People with diabetes should always carry glucose tablets (or plain hard candies) in case they need to raise their blood sugar quickly.

sugar. Even for someone who has his or her diabetes under control, illness, stress, eating too much of the wrong foods, miscounting carbs, or not taking enough insulin can cause high blood sugar, with some of these symptoms:

- Thirst
- Urination
- Fatigue
- Blurred vision
- Tingling in the feet or hands

Ketones

A person with type I diabetes routinely tests his or her urine or blood for ketones, the acidic product that results from the body burning fat, which happens when the body runs out of insulin.

People with diabetes used to test their urine for blood sugar, but this wasn't accurate and it couldn't measure low blood sugar. In addition to blood tests, people test for ketones by urinating on a ketone test strip or testing with a special meter that can test blood ketones.

The condition called ketoacidosis is very serious. Its symptoms usually begin with nausea, high blood sugar, feeling tired, having dry or flushed skin, vomiting, confusion, sweet fruity-smelling breath, and trouble breathing. Someone with untreated ketoacidosis may become sleepy, then unconscious, and possibly die.

Ketoacidosis is considered a medical emergency. If you have type I and the symptoms of ketones, you should test your blood immediately. If the ketone test is high, you need to call your doctor right away. Drinking many glasses of water will help flush the ketones out of your system, but you will also need insulin, possibly through an intravenous (IV) line.

Insulin

You will need to provide your body with a supply of insulin that matches what a healthy pancreas would produce—a steady amount, but with extra insulin at various times, especially at meals. The amount needed varies from person to person, and it changes for each person based on what and how much he or she is eating, what kind of exercise he or she is getting, and the person's stress level. It's a balancing act, and it takes people with diabetes and their support teams some time, patience, and experimenting to get it right.

Types of Insulin

Getting the right amount of insulin into the body has gotten easier in the last few years. There are now, for instance, insulins that begin working within five to fifteen minutes of when you take them, so that you can take them as you sit down to a meal. Even a few years ago, the insulin had to be injected thirty minutes to an hour before the meal. If a meal was delayed, the person's blood sugar level would drop through the floor.

Insulins begin acting at different speeds and work for different amounts of time. They also peak (have their greatest effect) at different times. Aside from the very fast-acting insulin, there are other options:

- Regular insulin, which begins working in thirty minutes to an hour, peaks at three to four hours, and lasts six to ten hours.
- Ultra-long-acting insulin (glargine and Levemir) starts working in a little more than an hour, but keeps working without peaks for twenty-four hours.

➤ Rapid-acting insulin (Novolog, Humalog, and Apidra) starts working in five to ten minutes, peaks in one-half or one hour, and lasts for about four hours.

Why so many types of insulin? Because it is tricky to adjust a person's insulin level as well as the pancreas does. Plus, a person with diabetes is trying to avoid "highs" and "lows" that fall outside of the target range: too much blood sugar makes it high, and too much insulin (from taking too much, or missing a meal) or misjudging exercise makes it low. A doctor will help determine a person's daily regimen—based on blood sugar levels—and adjust it. Often, two types of insulin are used, either in a combination shot or in several shots during the day. A combination of an ultra-long-acting insulin and a shorter-acting insulin (at mealtimes) more closely imitates the pancreas's output.

"Tight Control"

A study called the Diabetes Control and Complications Trial, conducted between 1983 and 1993, showed that people with type I diabetes who kept themselves more closely within blood sugar range had fewer long-term complications. The control group used the standard insulin therapy at that time, taking two shots a day and testing their blood two or three times during that period. The "intensive therapy" group tested themselves four to seven times a day, and either gave themselves three to four injections or used an insulin pump.

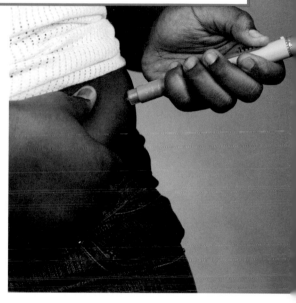

The insulin "pen" can be a convenient way to carry and inject insulin. Injections are the most common way people get insulin into their bodies.

They paid close attention to their blood sugar levels, aiming to keep these between 80 and 120 mg/dL, and adjusted their insulin to their blood sugar levels. This study proved conclusively that keeping the blood sugar in a nondiabetic range really made a difference in people's health, preventing the onset or the worsening of complications by 50 percent or more. (If that seems obvious or very late in medical history to discover this, then keep in mind that before this time there was no way to keep such close control over the blood sugar. Neither "real time" home blood tests nor the various kinds of insulin were available.) A more recent study shows similar results for people with type II diabetes.

Delivery Systems

Insulin must be injected into the body, or, with more recent technology, inhaled. Unfortunately, it cannot be taken as a pill because the process of digestion destroys it.

The most common way of injecting insulin is with a syringe: you have to give yourself shots in a fleshy part of the body like the stomach, arms, thighs, or buttocks. Easily transportable "pens" are available, so called because they are like fountain pens that hold insulin and have a needle attached.

There are also insulin pumps that are worn all the time and deliver insulin through a tiny tube inserted under the skin.

Making the Decision to Pump

Insulin pumps have become increasingly popular. They are as small as cell phones, or even smaller, and can be attached to a belt or waistband or hidden in a pocket. Inside the insulin pump are a container of insulin, a pump, and a tiny computer that is programmed to deliver insulin through a very skinny, flexible tube. You use a needle to insert the tube under your skin, and then remove the needle (as an IV is inserted in the hospital). Every few days you change the site, called the infusion site.

The pump delivers a preprogrammed dose of insulin. The mealtime extra dose, called a bolus, can be programmed into it or can be delivered by pressing a button. Some of the pumps are waterproof. They can be removed (without removing the delivery tube) for contact sports.

Many people who have switched to pumps feel they are great. The pump lets users increase dosages for meals easily and can deliver tiny, precise doses. You can change the hourly amount of insulin if you're sick or exercising a lot. They do away with the need for constant injections.

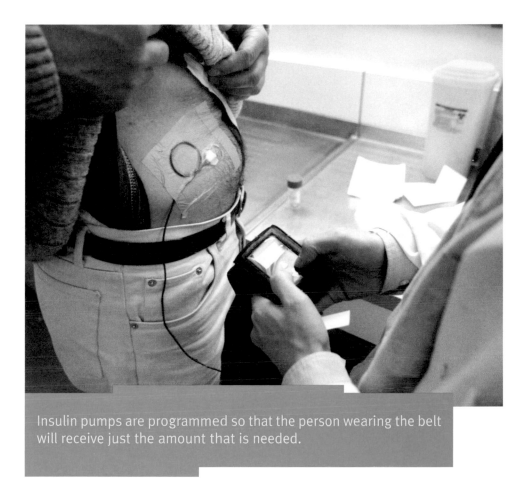

Insulin pumps are programmed so that the person wearing the belt will receive just the amount that is needed.

Some people dislike the idea of having a machine attached to their bodies all the time. The pump needs to be used correctly and monitored closely. Because it uses rapid-acting insulin, if the flow is cut off (and the pump's alarm system fails), the wearer could experience a problem with ketones quite quickly. The increased control over dose is useful only if a person is willing to test his or her blood often. There is some risk of infections at the infusion site. Pumps are also expensive.

Myths and Facts

About Diabetes

Myth **Diabetes is caused by eating too much sugar, and people with diabetes shouldn't eat sugar.**

Fact ➡ Diabetes is caused by too little insulin, not by eating too much sugar. In the past, people with type I diabetes were told not to eat sugar. Now, sugar is just one of the carbs that people with diabetes must keep track of. However, many people with diabetes feel that soft drinks, for instance, are just not worth the carbs.

People with a low blood sugar reading need sugar to get their blood level up. Taking glucose tablets (or an injection of glucagon for someone who is already unconscious) is the fastest way to return blood sugar level to normal.

Sugar by itself isn't the key issue for people with type II diabetes either. Their whole way of eating may be, though. If the body is having trouble using insulin, then keeping track of carbs and calories is important.

If type II diabetes isn't causing any problems, then it can be ignored until it acts up. Fact ➡ Diabetes complications take time to develop. It's incredibly hard to realize that something that isn't bothering you is really hurting you. It's also hard to realize that seemingly harmless behavior like not getting exercise, drinking soft drinks, and eating fast-food burgers often might give you a lifelong disease. Undiagnosed type II diabetes causes major health and quality-of-life problems, and its symptoms shouldn't be ignored.

Vanilla, cinnamon, aloe juice, chromium, or vitamin supplements can be used to control diabetes. Fact ➡ Juices and supplements have not been proved to control diabetes, though herbs and minerals are being studied as possibilities. If you hear about an alternative therapy, talk to your health team about it first. Supplements can interact badly with your medicines.

If you are interested in alternative healing practices, consider meditation or deep-breathing exercises. They can be great ways to handle stress, and stress can make diabetes (and the rest of life) harder to handle, as well as affect blood sugar levels.

Myth **Diabetes is contagious.** Fact ➥ You didn't catch diabetes from someone, and no one can catch it from you. If a blood relative has diabetes, there is a greater chance of you getting it. That's not because you caught it, but because a vulnerability to the disease can be inherited.

When many people in a neighborhood have type II diabetes, it is not because they caught it from each other, but because they share risk factors. These risk factors can include racial or ethnic backgrounds, eating and exercise habits, and lack of access to routine medical care.

The Combined Pump-Blood Monitor

In April 2006, the Food and Drug Administration (FDA) approved the first integrated insulin pump and continuous glucose monitor. An electrode inserted under the skin takes blood sugar readings every five minutes. Although glucose levels have to be confirmed by a fingerstick blood test (not every five minutes!), the constant monitoring allows people to correct out-of-range blood sugar almost immediately and spend far more time in range.

The Juvenile Diabetes Research Foundation (JDRF) called the new system an important step toward the development of an

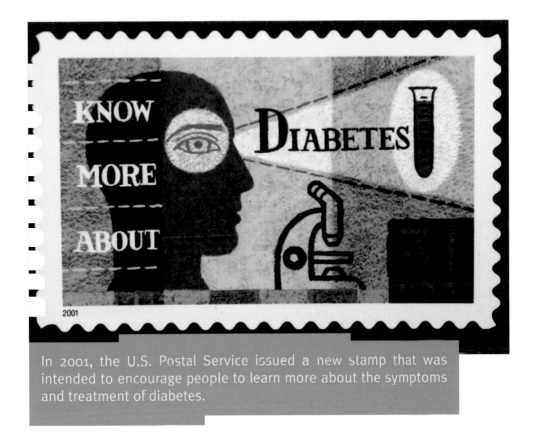

KNOW MORE ABOUT

DIABETES

2001

In 2001, the U.S. Postal Service issued a new stamp that was intended to encourage people to learn more about the symptoms and treatment of diabetes.

"artificial pancreas," which would test blood sugar as often as 1,400 times a day and deliver the correct amount of insulin automatically, as well as record glucose and insulin levels.

Type II Diabetes Medicines

For some people with type II diabetes, changing eating and exercise habits is enough to control the disease. Other people need to take pills. Some of the current medicines work to stimulate the pancreas to produce more insulin, decrease the body's resistance to insulin and use it better, slow down the process by which carbs are turned into sugar (which allows the body a longer time to absorb the sugar), or help the body be more sensitive to insulin so that less is needed for glucose to be absorbed by cells. These are different medicines, and a doctor may prescribe one or more of them.

If your pancreas isn't making enough insulin, or you aren't able to control your blood sugar with oral medications, then you may need insulin injections. Unlike people with type I diabetes, who must take insulin their whole lives (or until a cure is discovered), people with type II may use insulin for a short time and then stop using it.

HOW SHOULD I LIVE WITH DIABETES?

There are two important things to know about diabetes:

1. You don't have to go through this alone.
2. Although you should be getting a lot of help managing your diabetes, diabetes is a really serious invitation for you to take control of your own life.

Diabetes Team

You should have a "team" to help you learn how to take care of yourself. This might include your primary care doctor, an endocrinologist (a specialist in diseases of the endocrine system, of which the pancreas is a part), a diabetes educator, a dietician, a physiologist, an ophthalmologist (a different eye doctor from the one who checks if you need glasses), and a podiatrist (the eyes and feet of someone with diabetes

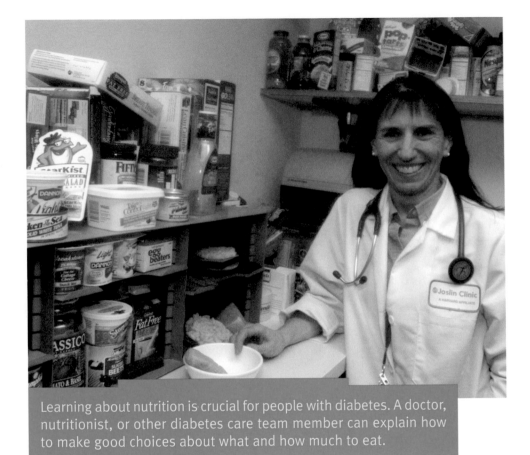

Learning about nutrition is crucial for people with diabetes. A doctor, nutritionist, or other diabetes care team member can explain how to make good choices about what and how much to eat.

are especially vulnerable to complications from high blood sugar). Other possible team members are social workers to help your family find resources (financial and emotional).

For many people, the diabetes educator is the member of the team who will help out with day-to-day living, including using medications, self-testing, record keeping, and handling high and low blood sugars.

Who Needs to Know About Your Diabetes?

Whom you tell about your diabetes is up to you. Some people make a point of pulling out their glucose meters on a first date. Others prefer to wait, feeling that no one needs to hear about their diabetes so soon. It's your choice. With that in mind, though, there are still some people who really do need to know, including your teachers and the school nurse, your coach, your boss, and your close friends, mainly the people who are around you regularly or are there to help you if you need it. When you test your blood or give yourself an injection in school, you don't need people calling the police. Your teachers need to know that you need a snack, no matter what the rules say about eating in class.

Having people around you who know can be a matter of comfort—you don't feel like you're keeping a big secret—and a matter of safety. If you become disoriented or unconscious from very low blood sugar (which can happen more quickly than a dangerous high), someone needs to know you need an emergency snack or a glucagon shot (if you're unconscious). You should have near you plain sugar candy or glucose tablets and an emergency glucagon kit.

Because of the danger of a "low" looking like drunkenness or drugs, it is also a really good idea to wear a medical ID, just as people with life-threatening allergies do. If you pass out or are in an accident, the ID alerts people taking care of you to monitor your blood sugar.

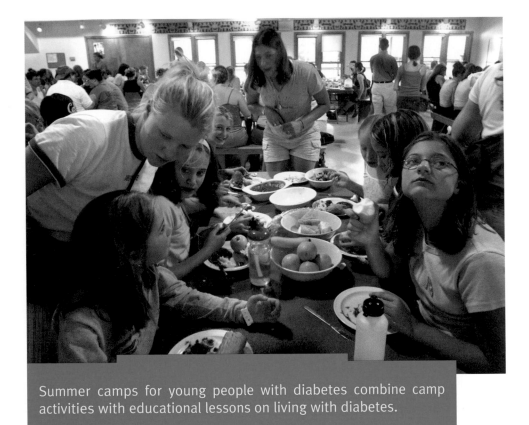

Summer camps for young people with diabetes combine camp activities with educational lessons on living with diabetes.

Support Groups and Online Chat Rooms

Your diabetes team may be able to help you find a local support group so you can talk to other teens.

There are also online chat rooms and message boards. On them you can howl with rage or compare notes about daily triumphs, frustrations, and insensitive classmates. They are a community of people who understand what you're going through and who may have a variety of ideas about how to handle some of the practical and emotional problems that will come up.

There are at least two things you should keep in mind when using a chat room or message board:

1. Don't change your treatment—food, exercise, insulin, or medications—based on advice you read anywhere on the Internet, including chat rooms.

   People may give advice that was good for them, but would be bad for you. They may, in fact, just give bad advice, even if that's not their intention. People's bodies process insulin at different speeds and need different amounts. If you hear about a product or a way of eating or anything that sounds interesting to you, ask your doctor or diabetes educator about it.

2. If you are not just mad or sad but really depressed, talk to an adult you trust. Diabetes may make you want to tear your hair out, but if it makes you feel that life is not worth living, you need some extra help coping.

Depression is more than just sadness. It can take away your energy and interest in the world. You may not be sad, just flat. If you are unable to sleep (or are sleeping all the time), have lost all interest in food (or are stuffing yourself uncontrollably), feeling hopeless, unable to concentrate, or unable to care about things you used to care about—don't deal with it alone and don't talk to people only in a chat room.

10 FACTS ABOUT DIABETES

1 In the United States in 2005, 20.8 million children, teens, and adults had diabetes—7 percent of the country's population.

2 About 14.6 million people have been diagnosed; an estimated 6.2 million have not.

3 Approximately 1.3 million people are diagnosed with diabetes each year.

4 More than 95,000 U.S. teens have type I diabetes.

5 About 39,000 U.S. teens have type II diabetes; 2.8 million teens are prediabetic.

6 One-third of people who have type II diabetes don't know it, and they may go seven to ten years without a diagnosis.

7 Eighty-two thousand amputations are performed each year on people with diabetes. Most of these could have been prevented through education and blood sugar management.

8 Diabetes was the sixth leading cause of death in the United States in 2002.

9 At least 171 million people in the world have diabetes. That number is expected to double by 2030.

10 Clinical trials show that with "tight" blood sugar control, most of the complications of diabetes can be prevented.

Diabetes Is Complicated Enough Without Getting Complications

Your doctors and diabetes educator are going to tell you that the way you take care of yourself will have a huge impact on the quality of your life now and later on. It's the truth. If you want to be well enough to go backpacking, have a job, party with your friends, or whatever, you need to keep your blood sugar under control, your eating habits healthy, and your body fit.

Your Eating Habits

Before accurate home blood testing and modern insulins, people with diabetes were severely limited in what they could eat. Sugar and most carbohydrates were generally forbidden. With modern testing and treatment, people balance carbohydrate intake with insulin and exercise. Carbohydrates are not just found in sweet breakfast cereal and cake, but also in breads, pasta, fruits, and vegetables. Somebody with diabetes can eat some of anything, but different amounts of various foods affect blood sugar. People with diabetes also need to get used to looking up the carb count of french fries, fry bread, rice and tofu scramble, and other foods.

People with diabetes are not on diets. Diets are what people go on for a while before they go back to eating "normally." What people with diabetes should be eating looks a lot like what everyone should be eating: a wide range of foods, including lots of veggies, whole grains, and proteins, and less fats, sweets, and white flour. With a diagnosis of diabetes, it becomes more important to eat better and—perhaps most of all—to understand what is being eaten. Skipping meals, going on fad diets, and indulging in mindless munchies go from being so-so options to being really lousy for the person with diabetes.

What You Eat Will Affect Your Health

A nutritionist or dietician should sit down with you and help you understand what you should be eating. Most people with diabetes realize that if they eat the same things at the same time each day, they don't have to think about their diet as much, but that is too restrictive and boring for most people.

The two main ways to organize your eating is by "exchanges" or by carb counting.

An exchange list is grouped by type of food: meats, starches, vegetables, fruits, milk products, and fats. You can trade or "exchange" items according to how many portions of each group you eat each day: one medium potato = $\frac{1}{2}$ English muffin = one carbohydrate exchange. The nutrition labels of many products list their exchange value.

Another way to keep track of what you're eating is to count carbohydrates. As forms of insulin have become more varied, it's easier for people with diabetes to count the number of carbohydrates in a meal or snack, and give themselves a dose of insulin that "covers" what they ate. However, a calorie is still a calorie when it comes to putting on weight.

If you have type II diabetes, then you and your nutritionist will probably design a way of eating that helps you lose weight. This helps your body use its insulin more efficiently and lowers the chances of your needing medicine—or insulin shots—as well as the dangers of complications. Carb counting will help you control your blood sugar but won't give you enough control over your weight.

Although the emphasis is on carb counting to control blood sugar, too much fat and cholesterol increase your chances of heart attacks and strokes later on—problems that are on the list of complications faced by people with diabetes.

Move It!

Physical activity is an important part of your treatment. Your muscles use glucose for energy during and after you exercise. Also, physical activity increases your sensitivity to insulin. What's more, exercise improves your circulation, helping prevent damage to nerves, and it naturally combats stress. Find exercises you like. Aerobic activities cause a sharper drop in blood sugar than

Some schools are encouraging students to get more exercise in order to lower their risk of developing type II diabetes.

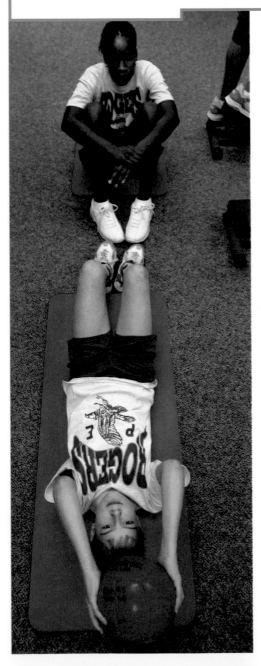

weight training or playing center field, so you should test your blood sugar more often if you're doing cardiovascular exercise.

Talk to your diabetes educator about how to exercise safely. Some of the advice you are given will be to check your blood sugar and for ketones in your urine before exercising. If your blood sugar is low, you should have a snack and then make sure it gets within range. If it's very high, above 300 mg/dL, you may be told not to exercise until you get it back down.

Real Life

When young children have diabetes, their families take

care of them. When you enter your teen years and want more independence, your parents may have trouble letting you take control. (You may, some days, not be so sure you want that responsibility either.) Control can be especially difficult during adolescence. As a kid, you may have had a regular bedtime and regular meal hours. Someone else was responsible for what you ate. As a teen, your school may have you eating lunch at a different time every day, you want to stay out late with your friends and then sleep as late as possible, and you just don't want to plan everything. You've probably got a lot of things that are more interesting to do than count carbohydrates. You probably don't want to be left out of activities or make a big deal about food and medical stuff with your friends.

You can do the things your friends do, if you plan for them. For instance, you can control your blood sugar during a long road trip by testing it before you drive and every two hours along the way. (Low blood sugar slows down reaction time, so it is really dangerous to drive with a low blood sugar.)

Other things your friends might do, you might want to reconsider.

Alcohol and Drugs

You can't legally drink alcohol if you're under twenty-one. If you have diabetes and drink, you are putting yourself at risk: alcohol can cause problems with your blood sugar. Don't drink on an empty stomach. It can also mask the signs of low blood sugar, since sounding "drunk" is one of the descriptions of low blood sugar.

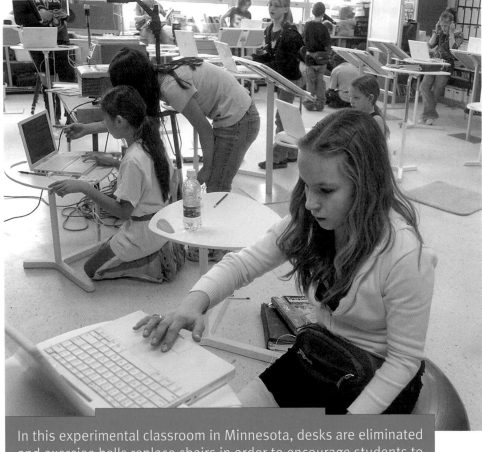

In this experimental classroom in Minnesota, desks are eliminated and exercise balls replace chairs in order to encourage students to move around, a way to incorporate exercise into the school day.

If you decide to drink despite the laws and the risk, then follow the advice given to adults with diabetes: limit what you drink (two drinks max), and don't choose drinks that are very sweet or very strong. Alcohol has calories and some carbs. Check your blood sugar frequently if you drink. If you drink be sure you are eating foods that contain carbs, and be careful with your insulin so that you don't get a low blood sugar. Keep your medical ID with you. Have not only a designated driver, but also a friend who will recognize if you have dangerously low blood sugar and who would know what to do about it.

Illegal drugs are likely to make you take less good care of your health. Even the munchies from marijuana can make your blood sugar run high. The stresses of living with diabetes make people wish they could just forget about it, and drugs might seem like they let you do that, but the risks are high. As with drinking, if you are going to take these risks, limit the danger to yourself as much as possible.

Tobacco

Aside from its other health risks, tobacco damages blood vessels. Since diabetes does, too, smoking or chewing tobacco increases your risk of high blood pressure and kidney disease.

Making the Most of Life

The hormones that are responsible for zits, beards, breasts, and other physical changes can make your insulin work less effectively. Hormone changes during adolescence usually mean more insulin is needed to keep your sugars under control. As you assume more responsibility for caring for your diabetes, work closely with your diabetes support team, your family, and close friends. If you've had diabetes since early childhood and have been in pretty good control, the blood sugar numbers may just seem bizarre. Sometimes, you're going to be out of target range. Although modern technology makes it easier to care for yourself, it still isn't easy. Don't kick yourself for "bad" numbers. Don't let an out-of-range number ruin your day. But in the long run, the cost of giving up and losing control is high. The payoff for taking control is that you can hope to avoid the scarier complications and do pretty much what you want with your life.

You might want to make diabetes a small part of your life. Or you might want to become involved in activities such as going to camp for kids with diabetes or becoming a counselor at one. Or, you may start a support group or raise money for diabetes research.

The bottom line is that diabetes makes life more complicated. There's no getting away from that fact. Yet as Olympian Kris Freeman discovered, diabetes didn't keep him from living the life he wanted. While diabetes certainly wasn't something Kelly would have chosen either, the challenge of not being limited by the disease actually led her to try new experiences that she otherwise might not have risked attempting. If you have been diagnosed with diabetes, you, too, can make the disease a small part of your life and make your accomplishments the main focus.

autoimmune disease Any disease in which the immune system attacks the body instead of infections and other invaders.

blood sugar The amount of glucose in the bloodstream.

bolus An extra dose of insulin taken before eating that takes the place of the insulin the body should be producing during and after a meal.

carbohydrates The sugars and starches that are consumed that the body turns into simple sugar (glucose), then energy. These include starches such as breads and cereals, rice and other grains, beans, potatoes, and corn; fruits; milk products ("lactose" is milk sugar); and vegetables.

diabetes mellitus The medical name for diabetes.

diabetic A term used to describe products designed for use by people with diabetes. It is sometimes used to describe people with diabetes, but many don't like the term since they feel it defines them by their disease.

diabetic ketoacidosis A dangerous level of ketones in the bloodstream caused by a lack of insulin.

dialysis The process of removing a patient's blood and running it through a machine for cleaning before returning it to him or her. This is necessary when the kidneys can no longer perform this function.

glucagon A hormone created by the pancreas that releases sugar stored in the liver into the blood. An injection of the hormone is the treatment for people whose blood sugar has fallen so low that they are unconscious or otherwise cannot swallow glucose tablets or gel or some other form of sugary snack.

glucose The simple sugar into which the body changes carbohydrates in order to use them for energy.

hemoglobin The protein that makes red blood cells red and carries oxygen through the bloodstream.

hyperglycemia Too much glucose in the bloodstream.

hypoglycemia Too little glucose in the bloodstream.

insulin One of the hormones produced by the pancreas. It allows cells to take in glucose from the bloodstream.

ketones The toxic acid produced when the body burns fats for fuel.

lancet A little needle, often set into an automated device, used to prick the skin to obtain a tiny blood sample for a blood glucose monitor.

pancreas The internal organ located behind the stomach that produces insulin and some other hormones.

American Diabetes Association
1701 N. Beauregard Street
Alexandria, VA 22311
(800) DIABETE (342-2383)
e-mail: askADA@diabetes.org
Web site: http://www.diabetes.org
  This is the largest nonprofit organization in the United States,
  focusing on diabetes research, advocacy, and education.

Canadian Diabetes Association
National Life Building
1400-522 University Avenue
Toronto, ON M5G 2R5
Canada
(800) 226-8464
e-mail: info@diabetes.ca
Web site: http://www.diabetes.ca
  This Canadian group promotes advocacy and education.

Centers for Disease Control and Prevention
1600 Clifton Road
Atlanta, GA 30333
(800) 311-3435
Web site: http://www.cdc.gov
  Part of the federal Department of Health and Human
  Services that focuses on public health issues.

Diabetes Exercise and Sports Association
8001 Montcastle Drive
Nashville, TN 37221
(800) 898-4322
Web site: http://www.diabetes-exercise.org
   An organization for people with diabetes (and also health
   care providers) who are interested in sports and exercise.

The Diabetes Monitor
51 Woods Road
Hillsborough, NJ 08844
e-mail: info@diabetesmonitor.com
Web site: http://www.diabetesmonitor.com
   This Web site provides information on medications and
   technological advances.

Juvenile Diabetes Research Foundation International
120 Wall Street
New York, NY 10005
(800) 533-CURE (2873)
Web site: http://www.jdrf.org
   This organization funds and reports on medical research and
   on the treatment and prevention of diabetes.

Web Sites

Due to the changing nature of Internet links, Rosen Publishing
has developed an online list of Web sites related to the subject
of this book. This site is updated regularly. Please use this link
to access the list

http://www.rosenlinks.com/faq/diab

American Diabetes Association. *American Diabetes Association Complete Guide to Diabetes Care*. 3rd edition. Alexandria, VA: The American Diabetes Association, 2002.

Betschart, Jean. *Type 2 Diabetes in Teens: Secrets for Success*. New York, NY: Wiley & Sons, 2002.

Betschart, Jean, and Susan Thom. *In Control: A Guide for Teens with Diabetes*. New York, NY: John Wiley & Sons, 1995.

Cairns, Douglas. *Dare to Dream: Flying Solo with Diabetes*. Boulder, CO: Albyne Press Ltd., 2005.

Collazo-Clavell, Maria. *Mayo Clinic on Managing Diabetes*. Rochester, MN: Mayo Clinic, 2001.

Kelly, Pat. *Coping with Diabetes*. New York, NY: Rosen Publishing Co., 2003.

Khalaf, Hala. *Young Voices: Life with Diabetes*. New York, NY: John Wiley & Sons, 2005.

Loy, Spike Nasmyth, and Bo Nasmyth Loy. *487 Really Cool Tips for Kids with Diabetes*. Alexandria, VA: The American Diabetes Association, 2004.

Loy, Spike Nasmyth, and Bo Nasmyth Loy. *Getting a Grip on Diabetes: Quick Tips & Techniques for Kids and Teens*. Alexandria, VA: The American Diabetes Association, 2000.

Moran, Katherine J. *Diabetes: The Ultimate Teen Guide*. Lanham, MD: Scarecrow Press, 2006.

Warshaw, Hope S. *Guide to Healthy Restaurant Eating.* 3rd
    edition. Alexandria, VA: The American Diabetes
    Association, 2005.
Wolpert, Howard. *Smart Pumping: A Practical Approach to the
    Insulin Pump.* Alexandria, VA: The American Diabetes
    Association, 2002.

Bibliography

American Diabetes Association. *Complete Guide to Diabetes Care*. 3rd edition. Alexandria, VA: The American Diabetes Association, 2002.

Betschart, Jean, and Susan Thom. *In Control: A Guide for Teens with Diabetes*. New York, NY: John Wiley & Sons, 1995.

Collazo-Clavall, Maria. *Mayo Clinic on Managing Diabetes*. Rochester, MN: Mayo Clinic, 2001

Kelly, Pat. *Coping with Diabetes*. New York, NY: Rosen Publishing, 2003.

index

About the Author

Judith Levin is a writer living in Brooklyn, New York. She has worked as a children's book editor and a children's librarian. She has written books about history and science for several presses. Levin became interested in the science—and challenges—of diabetes after several friends and family members of hers were diagnosed with the illness.

Photo Credits

Cover © Keith/Custom Medical Stock Photo, Inc.; p. 5 © Matthew Stockman/Getty Images; p. 9 © Birmingham/Custom Medical Stock Photo, Inc.; p. 11 © www.istockphoto.com/ Kenneth C. Zirkel; p. 12 © www.istockphoto.com/Monika Adamczyk; p. 16 Costin Cojocaru/Shutterstock.com; p. 17 © Ribotsky/Custom Medical Stock Photo, Inc.; p. 18 © GARO/ PHANIE/Photo Researchers, Inc.; p. 21 © Saturn Stills/Photo Researchers, Inc.; p. 24 © Cristina Pedrazzini/Photo Researchers, Inc.; p. 25 © Mark Harmel/Photo Researchers, Inc.; p. 29 © Leonard Lessin/Photo Researchers, Inc.; p. 33 © Coneyl Jay/ Photo Researchers, Inc.; p. 35 © Phanie/Photo Researchers, Inc.; p. 39 © U.S. Postal Service/AP/Wide World Photos; p. 42 © Angela Rowlings/AP/Wide World Photos; p. 44 © Michael Dwyer/AP/Wide World Photos; p. 50 © Eric Gay/AP/Wide World Photos; p. 52 © Janet Hostetter/AP/Wide World Photos.

Editor: Jun Lim; Designer: Evelyn Horovicz
Photo Researcher: Hillary Arnold